Aromatherapy

A Clinical Guide to Essential Oils for Holistic Healing

Table of Contents

Introduction

Science has recently been confirming what the ancients knew centuries ago - scents can have as much of an effect on our brains as the food we eat and other sensory inputs. A pungent scent may act as a warning that something is not good for us or that there is danger in the vicinity.

Scents are not always associated with warnings, however. Scents can also be associated with happy memories and the whiff of a familiar scent, associated with better times, is often enough to help lift one's mood. So it comes as no surprise to learn that smells can also help to relax or stimulate the brain and also to help us heal better.

According to the dictionary, the definition of "aromatherapy" is, "the use of natural oils that have a pleasant smell to make a person feel better especially by rubbing the oils into the skin."

The science of aromatherapy involves the derivation of the natural essences from various plants and the subsequent application of those essences in order to promote healing, both physically and mentally. This is an alternative form of therapy and can be considered quite safe – as long as you do your homework properly first.

Some of the gentler oils can be used by pregnant women quite safely and can provide an effective, curative treatment when conventional medicine is not deemed suitable. Essential oils can be used at almost every stage of your life, in order to help promote a healthier and happier you.

Over the course of this book, you will learn how you can use aromatherapy safely to best effective. We will go through the ten most popular oils, how to blend them together, how to safely apply them and what conditions they are best suited to treating.

Once you have worked you way through the whole book, you will be able to confidently mix and match oils to make effective treatments for you and your loved ones. You will learn how to create blends, store them and when and where to apply them.

Essential oils smell great and are great natural healers as well. They are a potent weapon in the fight against illness and can help to restore your vitality.

If you want to boost your health and help to fight off the effects of stress naturally, this book is going to be a real eye-opener for you. Not only will you learn how to use the oils, but I will also share some of my own special remedies with you - honed through many years of practical research.

Why don't we just jump right in then?

Chapter 1:
How Aromatherapy Works.

The Science behind Aromatherapy

If you want to truly understand why essential oils are so effective, it does make sense to understand a bit more about the chemistry at work. This will not only help you to improve your overall understanding but put you in much better stead when it comes to experimenting with your own blends.

Essential oils are natural but they still do have chemical components. This becomes very important when it comes to blending them properly. If you mix together two oils that have components that clash, the components work against one another, reducing the effectiveness of the blend as a whole.

The Chemical Make-Up of Essential Oils

By and large, the primary components of all essential oils are Carbon, Oxygen and Hydrogen. The differences between oils come in when we see how these components are combined and what ratios of each the oils have.

Most of the time, the essential oil consists of aromatic rings and a branched chain of around about five carbon compounds. It is in these rings that the scent of your essential oils is determined – the scent depends on the number of carbon atoms found in the rings. This can be as few as three or as many as five.

The actual components in the oil itself differ depending on the actual species of the plant, the growing conditions, where it is from and the method of extraction.

The Two Primary Essential Oil Compound Types

There are two main types when it comes to the basic compound types.

Terpenes: Terpenes are a big group of unsaturated, atomic hydrocarbons. What this boils down to is that they have space for more Hydrogen atoms in their make-up.

Oxygenated Compounds: It is these compounds that create the distinctive character of the oils. The term "oxygenated compounds" incorporates a large subset that includes ketones, aldehydes, alcohols, acids, phenols, coumarins, and esters.

For a blend to work well, each oil either needs to have a similar makeup in terms of each of these or at least needs to work well together with one of the others.

Knowing what the primary compound contained in the oil is also extremely important when it comes to safety. The furucoumarin, Bergaptene, for example, is one of the primary components in Bergamot oil. It is photo-sensitive, meaning that it reacts to U.V. light – if you go into the sun soon after applying this oil to your face, for example, it can cause the skin to darken or become irritated.

Compounds that May be Problematic

Ketones: Large concentrations of ketones can be problematic as they can irritate the skin. For best results, use very heavily diluted or use in a diffuser only

Phenols: Phenols can leave a residue in the liver and, if these oils are used on a regular basis, this can become toxic. It is important to ensure that you only use these for short periods of time and to ensure that there is a large rest period in between.

How Essential Oils Are Extracted

Essential oils can be sourced from many different areas in the plant. Generally speaking, the more fibrous the plant matter is, the harder the oils are to extract. Vertivert oil, for example, is extracted mainly from the roots and these need to be subjected to high pressure in order to squeeze out as much as possible.

Not all oils can stand up to rough handling though. In the case of Jasmine oil, for example, it is more common to make use of solvents to extract the oils as this is the more gentle process.

The price of oils can vary so much as to seem crazy – Rose Otto, for example, is ridiculously expensive and is out of reach for most budgets. Most of the rose essential oils that you see in the store will have been blended with something else because of the expense of producing the oils. It takes tons of rose petals to produce only a few pounds of essential oil and this makes it more expensive. On the other side of the scale, you have oils like Eucalyptus that are a lot less expensive to produce because the yield in terms of oil is so much higher.

Also, with roses, it is only the petals that can be used to extract the essential oils. Other plants, like oranges, are a lot more versatile – with oils being extracted from the leaves, flowers and the peel of the orange.

Essential Oils Year To Year

Much like a fine wine, essential oils can differ from one year to the next, depending on what conditions are present while the plants are growing. Whilst the species may remain the same, local weather conditions, harvesting methods, etc. all have a role to play in the quality of the oils produced. You'll get some good years and some less than good years as well.

This makes it even more important to choose a company that has built up a good reputation when it comes to the sourcing of essential oils. The experience of the wine-maker is important when it comes to wine but it is equally as important when it comes to essential oils.

The Different Forms of Essential Oils

"Essential oil" tends to be a term that is rather generally used to describe all kinds of natural, aromatic plant essences but this is not really accurate. Many of the processes used for the extraction of essential oils do leave a residue behind so you seldom get a "pure" oil. The method of extraction is important to ascertain because it can have a very real impact on the quality of the oils.

Oils derived from the flowers of plants, for example, need to be extracted fairly quickly after they are harvested. The roots and seeds, on the other hand, can hold up to being stored. The end quality of the oils does also depend on the quality of the plant matter used.

Essential Oils

There are two basic methods of extracting an essential oil – pressure or simple expression or through distillation – whether by water, steam or dry distillation. The more commonly available oils, like Sandalwood, Lavender and Cinnamon are generally extracted through steam distillation. This does, however, has its downside as only the parts of the plant that are not soluble in water are extracted, leaving some valuable components behind.

The oil may be run through a secondary distillation process in order to rid it of remaining impurities, etc. This process can be tweaked in order to reduce the amounts of undesirable components. Camphor, for example, can be distilled at three different levels – white, brown or yellow, by varying the heat used in order to effectively burn off remaining undesirable content.

For the most time, essential oils take a liquid form. This can vary to semi-solid, as is the case with Rose Otto, or solid. The oils are soluble in alcohol, oils and other fats but are insoluble in water. When they are exposed to air, they will simply evaporate and not leave a greasy residue behind.

Concretes

Concretes generally come from the vegetative parts of plants, such as the leaves, roots, herbs or flowers, rather than the fruits. These are extracted by means of exposure to solvents as opposed to steam or distillation and is necessary when the oil would be damaged if these processed were used. These oils will not stand up to heat or steam. The advantage of this method is that the oils extracted are as close to their natural scent as possible.

With some plant matter, like Clary Sage and Lavender, either method can be applied, depending on what the aim is at the end of the day.

Concretes typically have a ratio of half wax and half volatile oil. This can vary in special cases, such as in Ylang Ylang, where the ratio is a lot more weighted in favor of the oil.

Concretes are less volatile than the essential oils alone and tend to be more aromatic.

Resinoids

Resinoids must be extracted using a solvent like hexane or petroleum ether. Contrary to the case in concretes, resinoids are extracted from dead material, rather than material that was previously alive.

Balsams such as Benzoin or Peru Balsam are typical of the type, Amber and Mastic are examples of the resins, Turpentine and Copaiba Balsam are typical of the oleoresins; Frankincense and Myrrh are typical of the oleo gum resins. Resinoids can be viscous or solid but do tend to be thicker and more sluggish.

In some cases, the portion of the resinoid that is soluble in alcohol is referred to as an absolute.

Some resinous materials like Frankincense and Myrrh are used either to make an essential oil by steam distillation or a resin absolute by alcohol extraction directly from the crude oleo gum resin.

Benzoin, on the other hand, is not volatile enough to produce an essential oil by distillation: the Benzoin "essential oil" that you usually buy is quite often just the resinoid that has been dissolved in an appropriate solvent.

Resinoids, much like concretes, are a firm favorite in the beauty industry when it comes to fixing fragrances and making the last longer.

Absolutes

Absolutes are derived from the concrete through the use of solvents. Ethanol is the solvent of choice as the wax is largely insoluble in ethanol. The oil undergoes several exposures to remove as much of the wax as possible but a little will always remain.

The absolutes can then be subjected to molecular distillation in order to remove any left-over traces of non-volatile matter. Most of the alcohol evaporates leaving the pure oil but there is always the possibility that some traces can remain. Whilst these concentrations will be small, you should generally not consider these oils safe to use for therapy.

Much research lately has been put into using carbon dioxide to extract oils and it has been found that this is a far superior way to extract the oils.

Chapter 2:
Happy Families

The Basic Components of Essential Oils and How to Blend Them

In this chapter, we will go through the basic range of compounds within the essential oils and look at how t0 blend the oils in terms of these compounds and also in terms of the basic fragrance notes.

Plants produce compounds such as aldehydes, etc. in order to protect themselves from disease and to help them to thrive. These same compounds are what benefit us when we use the oils.

Each oil can contain hundreds of compounds so it is quite a complicated mix. In this chapter though, we will deal with the most common ones.

Where essential oils actually shine as a healing treatment is in their ability to easily pass through the skin barrier and to enter the blood stream. Alternatively, the compounds can be inhaled and enter the body through the lungs. In both cases, this makes uptake a lot faster than it would be through the digestive tract, making essential oils a much more effective delivery system.

The Science

We have already discussed the basics of the hydrogen, oxygen and carbon compounds so I am going to skip straight over to the compounds that interest us.

Terpenes

Common terpene hydrocarbons include limonene (antiviral, found in 90 per cent of citrus oils) and pinene (antiseptic, found in high proportions in pine and turpentine oils); also camphene, cadinene, caryophyllene, cedrene, dipentene, phellandrene, terpinene, sabinene, and myrcene among others.

Some sesquiterpenes, such as chamazulene and farnesol (both found in Chamomile oil), have been the object of great interest recently due to their outstanding anti-inflammatory and bactericidal properties.

Esters

Probably the most widespread group found in essential oils, which includes linalyl acetate (found in Bergamot, Clary Sage and Lavender), and geranyl acetate (found in Sweet Marjoram). They are characteristically fungicidal and sedative, often having a fruity aroma. Other esters include bornyl acetate, eugenyl acetate and lavendulyl acetate.

Aldehydes

Citral, citronellal and neral are important aldehydes found notably in lemon-scented oils such as Melissa, Lemongrass, Lemon Verbena and Citronella. Aldehydes in general have a sedative effect; Citral has been found to have specifically antiseptic properties. Other aldehydes include benzaldehyde, cinnamic aldehyde, cuminic aldehyde and perillaldehyde.

Ketones

Some of the most common toxic constituents are ketones, such as thujone found in Mugwort, Tansy, Sage and Wormwood; and pulegone found in Penny Royal and Buchu – but this does not mean that all ketones are dangerous. Non-toxic ketones include jasmone found in Jasmine, and fenchone in Fennel oil. Generally considered to ease congestion and aid the flow of mucus, ketones are often found in plants which are used for upper respiratory complaints, such as hyssop and sage. Other ketones include camphor, carvone, menthone, methyl nonyl ketone and pinocamphone.

Alcohols

One of the most useful groups of compounds, tending to have good antiseptic and antiviral properties with an uplifting quality; they are also generally non-toxic. Some of the most common terpene alcohols include linalol (found in Rosewood, Linaloe and Lavender), citronellol (found in Rose, Lemon, Eucalyptus and Geranium) and geraniol (found in Palmarosa); also borneol, menthol, nerol, terpineol, farnesol, vetiverol, benzyl alcohol and cedrol among others.

Phenols

These tend to have a bactericidal and strongly stimulating effect, but can be skin irritants. Common phenols include eugenol (found in Clove and West Indian Bay), thymol (found in Thyme), carvacrol (found in Oregano and Savory); also methyl eugenol, methyl chavicol, anethole, safrole, myristicin and apiol among others.

Oxides

By far the most important oxide is cineol (or eucalyptol) which stands virtually in a class of its own. It has an expectorant effect, well known as the principal constituent of Eucalyptus oil. It is also found in a wide range of other oils, especially those of a camphoraceous nature such as Rosemary, Bay Laurel, Tea Tree and Cajeput. Other oxides include linalol oxide found in hyssop (decumbent variety), ascaridol, bisabolol oxide and bisabolone oxide.

Blending Oils

If you are in a rush, stick to simple blends – oils that fall into the same family will mix well together. If you have a little more time, look for oils that have similar concentrations of the main ingredients listed above. Your camphoraceous oils such as those in the Myrtaceae group, such as Eucalyptus and Tea Tree oil, contain similar quantities of cineol, as do Rosemary and Lavender.

The fragrances from the floral families all tend to mix nicely together and so do the balsams, woods and citrus oils. Linaloe and Rosewood, for example, blend well together despite being from different families because they do contain similar proportions of linalol.

Then you have the superstars of the fragrance oils that seem to be able to mix with just about every other oil, to the benefit of both. Examples of these are Lavender oil, Rose oil and Jasmine oil. This makes them popular options in perfumery.

Certain combinations simply do not work – mixing any of the following three groups together results in an ineffective mix altogether as the compounds work against one another. The groups in question are Ketones (such as the Thujone present in Sage); Aldehydes (such as the Citronellal present in Citronella); and Phenols (Such as the eugenol present in Clove oil).

It isn't necessary to worry too much about what the components of the oils are when you are just starting out. What I advise is to start using the blends in this book until you are comfortable with blending oils – this will let you try the waters before you move onto making your own blends and help you in determining what a good blend smells like.

It is also advisable to look at what the basic benefits of the oils are before deciding to blend them together. Say for example, you take a calming oil like Roman Chamomile, it would be a mistake to blend it with an oil that is very stimulating like Rosemary because those two elements would work against one another. Start by looking for oils that have similar basic qualities to make a good blend.

Fragrance Families

I have listed the basic fragrance families at the end of this section. Whilst it is not a hard and fast rule that you must mix like with like, there are some combinations that work better than others. Citrus oils and wood oils are one such combination, as are citrus and spice oils.

In order to make a scent more interesting, you can add in notes that are completely opposite in terms of family. (As long as they will complement one another.)

Always be guided by your own personal preferences but do experiment as well. I have my favorite oils and oils that I really do not like – for example, I really dislike the green tones much. That said, I have found that some scents that I really do not like individually combine well to create a whole new, pleasant fragrance.

Green: Basil, Chamomile, Clary Sage, Eucalyptus, Galbanum, Pine, Rosemary, Spruce and Thyme

Spicy: Camphor, Fennel, Ginger, Juniper, Laurel, Sweet Marjoram, Myrrh, Tarragon and Tea Tree

Floral: Geranium, Jasmine, Lavender, Mimosa, Neroli, Rose, Rosewood, Violet and Ylang Ylang.

Citrus: Bergamot, Citronella, Grapefruit, Lemon, Lemongrass, Lime, Mandarin, Orange and Petitgrain.

Woody/ Balsamic: Ambrette, Angelica, Bay, Birch, Cedar Wood, Frankincense, Marigold, Patchouli, Sandalwood, Valerian and Yarrow.

Getting the Scent Right

Making the perfect scent is about more than just combining what looks good on paper. It does require careful attention to detail. Perfumery is a skill but it is something that you can hone over time. For your blends to be really effective, they should smell good as well and that is where it pays to spend a little more time experimenting. You want a scent that has different dimensions using oils that blend together seamlessly. Ideally, you should not be able to tell which exact oils were used, you should just be able to pick up some of the individual notes.

Commercial perfumes tend to be made up of a whole range of different components but at the heart of each are three or four main scents. Once the body of the scent has been composed, the scent is tweaked by adding small quantities of other scents to add more depth.

I advise starting out with no more than three scents initially, until you get the hang of things. It can be a bit overwhelming at first so keeping your blends simple is key. Once you become more confident in your blending abilities, you can start looking at adding in more oils – you will learn which basic blends work and which won't and can play around with mixing it up.

The Top, Base, and the Middle

The aim is to have a balanced scent and for this, you need to have three separate notes – a base note, a middle note and a top note. Each essential oil can be placed on one of the three categories, depending on how stable they are. Some oils, like Jasmine, can be placed in more than one category.

The Top Note: These notes are the lightest and most volatile. This is the scent that is apparent as soon as you open the bottle and the one that will last for the shortest period of time. Most of the citrus oils are top notes. Other top notes include Eucalyptus oil, Jasmine oil, Basil oil and Tea Tree oil.

The Middle Note: The notes have more body and staying power and will become apparent when the top note wears off. These oils are less volatile and will last longer. Many of the herbal oils can be classified as middle notes. Other middle notes include Lavender oil, Rosewood oil, Geranium oil, Sweet Marjoram oil and Rosemary oil.

The Base Notes: These are the notes that will come to the fore last of all but they are also the ones that will linger. These notes act as an anchor for the others, helping to preserve the scent longer. A lot of the wood and spice oils fall into the category. Other base notes include Rose oil, Patchouli oil, Benzoin oil, Jasmine oil, Myrrh oil, Vetiver oil, Sandalwood oil and Frankincense oil.

Ylang Ylang is in a class of its own here as it is considered to be a naturally balanced oil all on its own – it can be used as one oil that can fulfil each of the above-mentioned functions in a blend. It is considered a completely balanced oil.

When you start blending your oils, start with no more than a drop or two of each. Add your base note in first and then add in the others. Generally speaking you need to be a little more light-handed when it comes to the amount of the base note as these scents are so rich and deep that you risk overpowering the other scents.

When developing your own blends, add no more than a drop of oil at a time so that you can get the exact right, balanced scent.

Once you have your top, middle and base note and are happy with the combination, you can look at adding hints of other oils to increase the wow factor of the blend.

Write It Down Now

This is a really solid piece of advice but one that people tend to want to skip. I sometimes get so into the blending of the oils that I don't bother to write the mixture down – after all, I know I can remember what I put in. Except that it is hard to remember later on – I was messing around the one time and I hit upon a really great scent. I could have kicked myself for not making notes because I wanted to make more of it. The problem was that, though I could remember what oils I had used, I could not remember exactly how much of each oil that I used – and that was on the same day that I mixed the oils.

To this day, I regret not writing it down because I have not been able to recreate it. Who knows, it could have been the next Chanel No. 5 but alas it is gone forever!

Make a list of the oils that you put in and how many drops you add. I find that writing a simple list and writing a tick next to each oil to represent one drop of oil is a really quick and easy way to determine what should go into the oil.

Make some kind of record of it – you could even video all your blending sessions if you -want to. When you have time, transcribe everything into your own personal scent bible.

Take my word for it, no matter how enthusiastic you may be now, you will not be able to distinguish the quantities in the oils by smell alone later on – write it down. Even now, after all the years that I have been at this, I still battle to distinguish between more than two or three oils in a blend.

Writing the results of your experiments down will also help to prevent you from covering the same ground over and over again. Write down your recipes and label the bottles that you store your blends in for good measure.

Chapter 3:
Safety Information
READ THIS BEFORE YOU START USING THE OILS!

Aromatherapy Is Safe If You Follow the Rules

People make the mistake that because the oils are natural they are perfectly safe. What should be remembered though is that they are highly concentrated and, as with all things in life, there are some basic safety rules when using them.

Looking at that little bottle, it is hard to believe that it can be dangerous. Think of it this way – essential oils are similar to an herbal tea in a sense, except that they are about a thousand times as potent. Where you will use few tablespoons of the fresh herb to make a cup of tea, it will have taken several plants to make up one bottle of essential oils. Would you drink 100 cups of Chamomile tea a day?

Therapeutic Grade Oils

You will find that a lot of companies jump on the bandwagon when it comes to aromatherapy – you will find that a lot of hair and beauty products use the fact that they contain essential oils as a big selling point. Whilst these are very nice products for the most part, there is not a sufficient quantity of the aromatherapy oils in there to make a real difference.

The only oils that are suitable for use in healing are 100% pure oils. You can also buy pre-mixed oils that have been properly diluted but, again, you need to ensure that 100% pure oils are used. This might mean a bit of searching on your part but the effort will be rewarded when you begin to use the oils.

Most of the bigger grocery stores or drugstores will have a range of different essential oils on offer, at a range of different prices. It is important to choose a reputable brand that you can trust and not to simply buy the cheapest oil that you can find. Because you will only be using a few drops at a time, one bottle will last you a good long while so do consider buying one of the more expensive brands.

At the very least, use an established brand of oils. Using the really cheap blends can do more harm than good and my advice, if you are working on a tight budget, is to rather buy one or two of the quality brand of oils than stocking up with 10 of the cheapest brands. The really cheap brands are cheaper for a reason – either they are using a lower quality essential oil or they are watering the mix down with cheaper oils. Melissa oil, for example, is often diluted with Lemon Grass oil to keep costs down and, while they may smell similar, they have very different properties.

Look for oils that are labelled "100% Pure" or that are labelled "Therapeutic Grade". With the others, you may not even be getting what you think that you are. Good oils will also usually list the botanical and common names on the bottle. A really good oil will tell you what distillation method was used and what region the oils come from.

Where the Oil is from

Where the plants have been grown influences what components there are in the oils. A plant that is in a tough, arid environment will create a very different range of chemicals to protect itself. And the differences don't stop there – the storage of the plant matter and oils, how much rain the plants got and even the soil that the plants are grown in can all make a difference.

It is not necessary to make a federal case out of this though – if the company is a reputable one with an established track record, they probably have varied sources for the oils anyway and you are safe buying them.

The Extraction Process

Another way that the company can save money in producing the oils is in the extraction process. Solvent extraction is the least expensive method to use and will generally be the method of choice for the lower quality brands. The problem is that this is a short-cut and you can never really be sure how much residue is left in the oils themselves.

Water or steam distillation is a better way to do things for most of the high quality oils so it is a good idea to look for oils extracted by these means. As mentioned in previously though, not all oils can survive this extraction process – oils like Benzoin and Jasmine must be extracted with the use of solvents.

Fragrance Oils and Blends

Fragrance oils are meant to be just that – for fragrance. They should never be used for healing though. In fact, as far as I am concerned, they should be avoided altogether. They are completely synthetic and could actually harm your health.

Blended oils are not always bad, as long as you know what you are getting in the blend. It is common practice to mix the more expensive oils with less pricey ones in order to bring down the price but a reputable company will always mark these oils as blends and list the other oils in the mix.

Rose oil, for example, is often bulked out with Rose Geranium oil and, if you know this, you can work around it. Problems crop up when the company does not list the oils in the blend.

You Get What You Pay For

I am not saying that you need to buy the most expensive oils on the market but you should look to price as an indicator of quality. As mentioned before, some oils require a lot more plant matter in order to get the oils needed. Some oils are sourced from rarer plants and so, naturally some oils will cost more than others. If you find a brand where the prices are pretty much the same across the board, or where the prices are a whole lot less expensive, do take care. If the Jasmine oil costs the same as the Eucalyptus oil and is not marked as a blended oil, the company is not being honest as regards its products and should not be supported.

The Right Dilutions

With the exception of Tea Tree oil and Lavender oil, oils should never be applied neat. Apart from these two oils, ALL the other oils are too concentrated to apply undiluted. If you use them in this manner, you risk burning your skin or causing irritation.

A simple rule of thumb is to dilute all oils before applying them – even if you are adding them to your bath water.

It is also important to use concentrations appropriate for the condition being treated and the age of the person that is being treated.

Oils used for children should always be heavily diluted and should be used in smaller quantities. The same goes for oils used on the sick or very frail. (Oils can have powerful detoxifying effects and this can cause problems for those who are weaker.

I find that it is a good idea to make up blends that I use on a regular basis and just keep them at the ready for when I need them – that way dilution is not as much of an issue.

Small Children and Animals

You need to always keep your oils out of reach of young children and animals. I once had a harrowing afternoon after finding that my dog had gotten hold of the Tea Tree oil and chewed the lid off. I still don't know whether or not he ingested any – taken internally, these oils can be toxic. I learned my lesson though and keep the oils out of reach.

I also had a friend whose little three-year old got stuck into her bottle of essential oils. He managed to open all the bottles and, when she got to him, he had poured the oils onto the floor and was playing splish splash. Fortunately he didn't drink the oils and she managed to wipe off most of it before it burned his skin.

If your child does get the neat oils onto themselves, remove using a wet facecloth. You can dampen the facecloth with water or milk. Apply baby bum cream or aqueous lotion afterwards to help soothe the skin and prevent further irritation.

If the oils get into any of the mucous membranes or eyes, apply milk – water will just make the problem worse as the oils will not dissolve in it. Once you have rinsed the oils out with milk, use lukewarm water to clean off the excess.

If you think your child swallowed the oils or if it looks like the skin is burned, get them to a doctor immediately.

Internal Use

There is a whole branch of French aromatherapy that advocates using the oils internally. This is always done under the control of a trained therapist though and should not be attempted at home. Not only can the oils be poisonous if swallowed – 4ml of Eucalyptus oil, for example will kill you if taken internally, but, even when used in small quantities, they can leave a residue that can build up to toxic levels in the bloodstream.

NOT for Newborns

Aromatherapy is suitable for most stages in life, the exception being babies who are less than 10 weeks old. At this stage in an infant's life, you could cause long-term sensitivities to the oil in question because their immune systems are not yet fully developed.

At 10 weeks, you can use a gentler oil such as Roman Chamomile oil or Lavender oil, as long as it is well diluted. Always do a small patch test on the baby's skin before slathering them in oils.

If you have any doubts as to whether or not baby's skin is too sensitive for the oils, you can always use them in a diffuser instead. Monitor baby to see what their reaction is to this diffusion of oils. If you see any signs of discomfort, get them out of the room straight away.

Don't Ignore Proper Dosage

Your child's size and age should be a factor when determining what dose of oils to use. Generally speaking, the smaller the child, the smaller the dose should be. Generally speaking, the oils should not be more than 0.5% - 1% of the overall total.

Photo-Toxic Oils

Some oils, particularly citrus oils, are photo-toxic. This is not as bad as it sounds, all it means is that the oils will react to the sun or UV light and that this can sensitize the skin, cause discoloration or a rash. If you are using these oils, ensure that the treated skin will not be exposed to sunlight for at least an hour or two.

Store Properly

In order for you to get the results that you would like from your aromatherapy projects, it is important to ensure that the oils are stored properly. This also applies to the carrier oils that you are using.

You need to keep the oils out of direct sunlight and away from direct heat, preferably somewhere that has an even temperature.

Before putting the oils away, do make sure that the bottles are properly screwed shut to avoid air getting in.

Beware of Rancid Oils

Essential oils are not really oils at all but they will also not last forever. Stored properly, some oils can be safely used up to around 2-3 years after being opened. Citrus oils like Lemon, for example, are a notable exception here and can go off in about 6 months.

Keep it simple for yourself and just enough oil to last around about 6 months.

The carrier oils that you use can also go rancid – work on a period of around 6 months to 2-3 years. Avocado oil, for example, will go off more quickly than Grape Seed oil. I always buy smaller bottles of specialist oils like avocado because I know that I will not use as much of them.

When oils are blended together, the blend will usually have a lifespan of around 6 – 12 months overall. Oils like Sandalwood and Cedar Wood can be added to the blend to help fix the fragrance. When making a blend though, I find that it is always better to make it up as you need it. I use smaller bottles that can be used within 2 – 3 weeks to be on the safe side.

With both essential oils and carrier oils, changes in smell, color and texture are indicative that the oil is past its expiry date and should be thrown out. Using rancid oils will end up being a waste of time at best and can cause irritation or sensitization at best so don't take a chance - if in doubt, throw it out.

Keep it Simple

It is tempting to throw together a whole bunch of oils in order to get the best benefit. As long as you check that the oils will all work in synergy with one another, you can add as many oils as you like.

I do advise to stick to no more than 6 oils in any one blend. Over and above that, it starts to get difficult to ensure that the oils all work well together and the blend can become too complex.

Ordinarily, you will know straight away if you have messed up with the blending because the oils will not smell good.

When you are trying out a new oil or a new batch of oils, I advise using it by itself to ensure that it does not cause any adverse reactions. If, for example, you blend together 6 oils and have an adverse reaction, it will be a lot harder to establish which of the oils caused the problem.

Once you have firmly established that the oils are not going to cause an adverse reaction, you can start experimenting and adding more oils to the mix.

Label Everything

I used to buy glass jars for the blends I made at the dollar store. This was great, until I started having a few different blends lying around. I suggest that, in addition to writing down your recipes, you also ensure that you either number or name the blend and then label the bottles accordingly.

I always put the labels on the top of the lids, where they are less likely to have oil spilled on them – the oil makes the labels illegible. Alternatively, attach the labels to the side of the bottle and cover them completely with clear adhesive plastic or cello tape so that none of the paper is uncovered.

Once again, make sure to do this as soon as possible after blending. You will often make blends that smell very similar to one another and it is not always possible to identify the blend through smell. I have wasted a lot of oils because I did not write out labels and could not remember what happened to the labels.

Patch Tests

Patch tests are important when using a new blend. If the oil irritates your skin, you will need to either dilute it more or to scrap the blend and try again. The more sensitive your skin, the more careful you need to be when it comes to diluting the oils and to what oils you actually use.

I do patch tests whenever I either try out a different oil or buy a new bottle of oils as one batch can differ from the next. It is also important to check that the oils have not gone rancid if you have not used them in a while.

Glass is Better

Glass is a better bet than plastic when it comes to making up blends. I also use the thick plastic containers from my prescription medications for smaller quantities from time to time but I do prefer using glass.

Glass bottles can be washed in soapy water and reused. This is more difficult with plastic bottles as the oils can actually interact with the plastic and degrade t.

Baby food jars make nice alternatives to buying new jars as long as they are properly washed and aired first. Any glass jar will do, as long as long as there is not lingering scent of food in it.

If you are making up a blend for a once-off use, plastic is okay. If you are making a blend for longer term use, glass is far better.

Once you have used a glass jar to store a blend in, it is no longer suitable to use to store food in.

Look for bottles that have lids that fasten securely and ensure that the bottle will work for whatever you are making. If you are making a body butter, for example, you need a shallow, wide-mouthed jar so that you can scoop it out easily. If you are making an oil blend, it is better to have a narrow necked jar so that you can better control the dispensing of the oil.

Begin with the Lowest Concentration

We always tend to think that bigger is better. It is very tempting to add in more oils because we think that this will create a stronger effect.

I always advise starting at the lowest dilution and working your way up only of that is not effective.

The stronger the concentration of oils, the higher the chance of causing irritation to the skin and the greater the chance of toxic residues building up. It is also possible for your body to get used to the effect of the blend over time and so it is better to use smaller concentrations at first and bump them up if you start to develop a tolerance.

Another possible concern is that too high a dose can lead to sensitization and you could end up developing an allergy to that particular oil.

The good news is that, even in lower concentrations, essential oils are highly effective.

Chapter 4:
The Therapist's Cheat Sheet

The Top 10 Most Useful Oils

There are literally hundreds of oils that you can choose from and it can be a bit of a problem deciding which ones to buy initially. It may be tempting to buy a whole bunch of different ones but this is not necessary.

You Should Like the Smell

Everyone has their own personal preferences when it comes to scents. If there are testers that you can use to test the oils before buying, I advise that you use them to see which scents you like.

The simple fact is that you will not use oils that you do not like and, if you buy them, no matter how beneficial they are, they will end up languishing in the back of the closet. I really dislike the smell of Tea Tree oil, for example, and I did buy a bottle of it but it was a waste of money because I really only use it now for making my dog's shampoo.

If you like one scent in a particular family of scents, for example, Sandalwood, there is a good chance that you will like other scents in the same family as well, like Cedar Wood, for example.

Almost a Never-Ending Story

Because of the quantities that we are dealing with, one small bottle is going to last you a long time. Choose two to three to start off with and see how you go. You can always add more later. Whilst it is nice to have a larger range of oils to choose from, it can actually end up being wasteful.

The Top 10 Most Useful Oils

These are the top 10 oils most useful oils. The first three are pretty much essentials, you can add to these as you wish.

Lavender

I always say that if you can only choose one oil, this is the one to get. Lavender blends with just about every other oil and smells wonderful. It is the most versatile of all the oils when it comes to healing properties. Lavender is also one of the most popular oils world-wide.

It is gentle enough to be used neat where necessary and can be safely used on infants from the age of 10 weeks onwards. Your furry friends can also benefit from the use of Lavender oil as it helps to repel ticks and fleas – it is safe for both dogs and cats.

If you have little children or like to garden, Lavender oil should have a place in your first aid kit. Make up a blend with Grape Seed oil to keep on hand to deal with minor scrapes and scratches, itchy bites, rashes, grazes, burns and bruises.

It can help to cure infectious skin ailments like chicken pox and ringworm and promotes the healing of the skin. Mixed with a bit of full-fat milk, it makes a great soother for sunburn. Mixed with a bit of apple cider vinegar, it makes and effective lice treatment.

It helps to take the sting out of burns and cuts and can help reduce the swelling, redness and itchiness associated with allergic rashes. It is a potent anti-bacterial and anti-viral agent and has strong anti-fungal properties as well. It is a great skin rejuvenator.

Used in a diffuser it can help soothe a chesty cough and clear up colds and flu, making breathing a lot easier. It can also help to soothe troubled nerves, encourage a restful sleep and calm anxiety.

Apply a drop to each temple and massage in when you have a headache to ease it.

Do the same when you have a migraine and also make a cold compress to place at the back of the neck using a few drops of the oil in a bowl of water. Nausea associated with the migraine can be eased by rubbing Lavender oil over the tummy area.

Add a few drops of the oil to your bath water at night to help ease stiff and sore muscles. Make a blend in a carrier oil to massage directly into the muscles as a follow up treatment.

If you do have trouble falling asleep, diffuse some Lavender oil in your room for at least half an hour to help you drop off or put some drops of the neat oil on your pillow.

You should have no trouble finding Lavender oil and will find that it is reasonably priced. It is usually used as a Middle note and is very easy to blend with other oils. It has an herby scent.

Eucalyptus Oil

If you love playing sports or competing in athletics, you need to add this oil to your first aid kit. It is a great treatment for tired and strained muscles.

If you or anyone in the home picks up colds and flu quite easily, this oil is also essential. It will blend with Lavender oil to make a potent cold and flu treatment.

The scent is best described as clean and clinical and it can be quite strong. The oil itself had great anti-bacterial and anti-viral properties. It can clear up congestion in minutes when diffused into the room and will help reduce the severity of a sinus headache. If you have a cold or flu, rub a mixture of Lavender oil and Eucalyptus oil into the soles of the feet and your chest last thing at night to help fight off the infection and to help reduce a high fever.

It can be applied to the skin in diluted form to help treat skin infections. Do dilute well though as it can irritate the skin.

A eucalyptus candle burned outside can help to repel insects on a hot summer's night.

You can make a very effective cellulite treatment by blending a few drops of Eucalyptus oil and Juniper oil into a paste of used coffee grounds and water. Massage onto affected areas, leave for a few minutes and then rinse off with warm water.

It is classified as a Top note when it comes to blending - meaning that the scent is one of the more volatile ones. It can be blended with Basil, Benzoin, Cedar Wood, Frankincense, Juniper, Lavender, Lemon, Marjoram, Melissa, Rosemary and Thyme.

Roman Chamomile

Roman Chamomile oil is an extremely useful oil that is essential if you have a young child. The scent is quite sweet but not at all overpowering and it can be used from the age of 10 weeks on.

It is when it comes to pain-relief that this oil really shines. It is the best analgesic out of all the oils. Mix with Lavender oil to help cure a headache – add it to a cold compress and apply to the back of the neck. Mix into a carrier oil for a great treatment.

If you have a bad tooth ache, or when you little one is teething, Chamomile will provide effective pain relief and will ease the throbbing ache. Ramp up its analgesic properties by creating a blend of Lavender and Chamomile and apply to the outside of the affected area. A couple of drops of the same blend dropped into the ear can help clear an ear infection.

It is great at soothing stress and anxiety and can stop a temper tantrum in its tracks.

In addition to its analgesic properties, it is also a very effective anti-inflammatory.

As an anti-spasmodic, it can be used to ease an upset tummy or to soothe menstrual pains.

It can help to soothe allergic skin reactions and eczema. It helps to soothe dry, troubled skin - mix with Lavender and Sandalwood for a wonderful treatment for skin that is suffering from exposure.

It is classified as a Middle note and will blend well with Benzoin, Bergamot, Clary Sage, Geranium, Jasmine, Lavender, Marjoram, Melissa, Patchouli, Rose and Ylang Ylang.

Sandalwood

Sandalwood oil is one of the more expensive oils but a little really goes a long way. It is a superb fixative oil and blends well with many different oils. I have to admit that this is one of my favorite oils. I also find that I use it a lot. If the cost is too much for you, Cedar Wood oil has similar properties but is more affordable.

Sandalwood is particularly important if you have mature, dry skin. Mixed into a blend of Neroli, Palmarosa and Lavender, it is a potent anti-wrinkle treatment to use at night.

It is a great sinus cleanser and will help alleviate dry coughs and the symptoms of colds and the flu.

Where it really shines though is in its ability to help you to relax and relieve nervous tension, especially when these are a result of a fear of change.

As a fixative, there is no oil to match it. I once made a batch of aqueous cream, using Sandalwood as the fixative and no preservatives. The bottle rolled under a bookcase and I forgot about it. A couple of years later, we moved house and the bottle was found. The blend still smelled as good as it had on the day it was blended.

Neroli

I love the smell of Neroli oil - it smells great and is a wonderful addition to any perfume blend.

Just a note of caution here though - when I was still working, a friend of mine and I decided that we needed a bit of a pick-me-up. We took a piece of cotton and added a few drops of Neroli. This we then put onto the radiator. The warmth from the radiator heated the oils and the scent permeated the room and very soon we were feeling great. We added a few more drops. After about an hour though, we were feeling a little too high-spirited and found just about everything funny. We had developed a mild buzz just from the Neroli oil! Granted, the room we were working in was pretty small and we had the windows closed to keep warm but this was one occasion when we had too much of a good thing.

If you are using the oil in a diffuser, make sure to use it for about a maximum of half an hour at a time. Alternatively, make sure that the room is properly ventilated. In all fairness, this never happened again and I use Neroli oil quite often in my perfume blends.

If you have a scar or stretch marks, this is a great oil to have on hand - blended with Lavender and Geranium and Rosehip oil, this is a wonderful treatment oil to encourage the reduction of scar tissue and to help regenerate skin.

Combined with Sandalwood it makes a perfect treatment for dry or dehydrated skin.

If you are battling with poor circulation, this is a good oil to use. It also has anti-spasmodic properties so can help relieve cramping.

If you have chronic diarrhea or flatulence, rubbing a Neroli blend into the abdomen can provide much needed relief. It is particularly helpful in treating Irritable Bowel Syndrome.

It is a very uplifting oil and is effective in treating depression and nervous tension. Use a blend of Neroli when you are feeling especially anxious and it will calm you down very quickly.

Perhaps I am just biased because I love the scent of Neroli oil but it is one of the best oils for perfume. It is a citrus oil but does not smell overtly of citrus - to me it is more floral and sweet. It provides a great top note for a perfume blend. It blends well with most other oils but is especially good with Benzoin, Frankincense, Geranium, Lavender and Rose.

Geranium

This is another of the oils that I always keep on hand. It is an inexpensive oil that is really great for the skin and so I often use it in blends. It is often used in Rose blends as it has similar properties to Rose oil and is said to smell like Rose oil. (Personally, to me it smells very different from Rose - it has a very herbaceous aroma.)

This does tend to overpower blends so I use 2 drops of any other oils in the blend for every 1 drop of Geranium oil.

The oil is a powerful skin healer and regenerator. For a particularly effective eczema treatment, get yourself an organic aqueous cream, some Geranium oil, some Palmarosa oil and Sandalwood oil. Used twice daily, this will clear up eczema and other allergic skin reactions.

There are no oils to beat Geranium when it comes to skin treatments - it helps to balance troubled skin and hydrate dry skin. Use on sunburned skin to reduce blistering and to soothe the burn. Apply to insect bites and allergic rashes for instant relief.

It is a good anti-inflammatory and so will reduce the appearance of red, raised pimples, prevent the infection of these, promote healing and reduce the chances of scarring.

I always mix up a bit of Lavender and Geranium oil whenever I am planning to do some crafting - it can be applied to cuts (my rotary cutter also hates me) and burns and will help them heal faster.

If you battle with water retention or cellulite, mix a few drops of oil into some olive oil and enough coarse salt to make a paste. Apply to the areas worst affected and then rinse off in a warm shower or soak off in a warm bath. Skin will feel smoother and softer and circulation will be boosted.

Geranium oil is said to have a balancing effect on the hormonal system and so can be useful if you suffer with premenstrual syndrome or if you are menopausal.

This is an uplifting oil that is useful in the treatment of depression and nervous tension.

It should not be used by pregnant women in their first trimester and should not be used by those diagnosed with breast or ovarian cancer.

This is classified as a Middle note and blends well with Basil, Bergamot, Grapefruit, Jasmine, Lavender, Neroli, Orange, Patchouli, Petitgrain, Rose, Rosemary, Sandalwood, and Ylang.

Ylang Ylang

If you want an oil that is truly exotic, this is it. You are either going to love it or hate it, there is no middle ground here. I love it but use it in limited quantities as it has quite a heady scent. If I feel a headache coming on, I avoid it as the strong scent can make a headache worse.

It is useful in balancing the sebum levels in the skin - making it suitable for use by people with all types of skin. Used in the rinse water after shampooing your hair, it helps increase shine and healthy hair.

It can be helpful at reducing high blood pressure and at regulating the heart.

It helps to reduce nervous tension and is renowned as an aphrodisiac. It can help to treat insomnia but I find that you need to be careful to use it in a blend here as the scent alone can end up being too strong. (I once sprinkled a few drops on my pillow to help me to sleep only to find that I needed to swap out my pillow because of the scent.)

What I find more effective is to mix 1 drop of Ylang Ylang, 1 drop Vetiver and 2 drops of Sandalwood and put them in the diffuser half an hour or so before bedtime. This is a very relaxing blend.

What I really love Ylang Ylang for is as a perfume oil - it rounds off sharp notes and can really take your perfume blend up to the next level. It also acts as a fixative in perfumes.

This is classified as a Base note and blends well with Grapefruit, Bergamot, Orange, Jasmine, Geranium, Sandalwood and Vetiver.

Sweet Marjoram

This is not an oil that is commonly recommended in popular magazines, etc. and I think that this is such a pity. Whilst this is not an oil that I would use in perfumery because it has a strong scent, I do find that its other qualities more than make up for this.

I find that it is particularly useful for relieving tired and sore muscles and joints, especially if blended with a little Lavender oil. It warms the muscles and is very soothing overall.

If you battle with circulatory problems or high blood pressure, this is one oil that should be on your shopping list - it can help reduce bruising, regulate blood pressure and also prevent chilblains.

It has strong anti-bacterial and anti-viral properties making it useful in the treatment of colds and the flu. Mixed with Chamomile and Lavender oils, it makes a soothing rub for a tight chest and wracking cough.

It has anti-spasmodic properties and can be used in a warm compress to help alleviate menstrual cramps and pain. It helps to regulate the menstrual cycle, particularly when blended with Clary Sage.

For me personally, it is its calming effect that is most helpful. If I find that I am feeling panicky or over-anxious, Sweet Marjoram blended with either Lime or Chamomile always helps me put things back into perspective.

Mixed with Lavender and Chamomile, this makes a really effective treatment for headaches and migraines - massage into the temple or use as a cool compress over the forehead and at the back of the neck.

Peppermint

I'm pretty sure that you have heard about the digestion soothing effects of Peppermint tea. The essential oil is equally as useful but also has a few uses that you may not have known about.

Peppermint's regulating effects on the digestive system make it a truly useful herb and one that does deserve a place in the top ten. It can help to ease dyspepsia, indigestion, colic and flatulence.

It also has strong anti-spasmodic properties making it a valuable addition to a post-workout blend. In addition, is aids circulation, warms muscles and soothes aches in muscles and joints.

I do avoid using the oil on my face though and do only use it at a maximum of 1% dilution as it may cause irritation to the skin.

I find that the oil is especially useful in the treatment of head colds - there is nothing better to clear up a nasty sinus infection than a blend of Peppermint, Eucalyptus and Lavender oils.

I use this oil a lot when I need to focus - it is a very stimulating oil and clears out foggy thinking very fast. It should not be used near to bedtime as it can keep you awake.

It can also interfere with the efficacy of homeopathic treatments and should never be used by pregnant women.

Rosemary

Rosemary is another of those scents that you will either love or hate. It is quite a strong scent and can be overpowering in a blend so again, use 2 drops of your other oils with every 1 drop of Rosemary oil.

This is one oil that is very good for oily skin and is useful in the treatment of acne. It is too harsh for dry or sensitive skin though. It is a great oil to help stimulate hair growth - rub a blend of Rosemary and Lavender into the scalp just about half an hour before washing your hair to help promote hair growth and a healthy scalp. (Preferably not within 2-3 hours of bedtime).

It is a very effective stimulant for the circulatory system and warms muscles. It has analgesic properties so is particularly good for those suffering from muscle stiffness and soreness, especially when this is due to overwork. It can also be valuable in relieving arthritic and rheumatic pain.

Rosemary oil is a good tonic for the liver and gallbladder so rub over the abdomen after over-indulging.

Rosemary oil is very effective at treating disorders of the respiratory system such as sinusitis and bronchitis. Blend with eucalyptus to ease coughing and wheezing.

Rosemary is also very useful in the treatment of headaches, especially if these are brought on by stress and tension. Apply as a cool compress to the back of the neck.

In ancient times, Roman soldiers would tuck a sprig of Rosemary behind their ears to help them focus their attention. This tactic is just as effective when using Rosemary oil. When I really need to focus on writing or studying, I blend together Rosemary oil and Lime oil and massage it into my scalp. I find that this helps me to focus for longer periods of time and lets me work longer and harder, with less chance of fatigue setting in.

Rosemary is classified as a Middle note and blends well with Basil, Bergamot, Frankincense, Geranium, Grapefruit, Lavender, Lemongrass, Lime, Mandarin, Orange, Pine and Petitgrain.

These are the 10 oils that I find most useful. With the exception of the first three, which should be part of every essential oil first aid kit, I encourage you to pick and choose oils that you think will be most useful to you.

Start off with the three essential oils and see how that goes. If you enjoy practicing aromatherapy, add a few of the other oils in the list. There is no rush to build up the ultimate collection of oils - add them as and when your budget allows you to.

Here is a quick break down of which oils to use for what (there may be some overlap - some oils fall into several categories:

Analgesics: Analgesics relieve pain. Good oils in this category include Peppermint, Black Pepper, Chamomile, Sweet Marjoram, Rosemary and Juniper. Clove can also be used if well-diluted and in moderation.

Anti-Inflammatory: Anti-inflammatory oils reduce swelling. Good oils in this category include Eucalyptus, Peppermint, Tea Tree, Chamomile, Lavender, Frankincense, and Myrrh.

Antiseptics: These oils clean wounds and help to prevent infection. Good oils in this category include Bergamot, Tea Tree, Lemon, Lavender, Rosemary, Thyme, Frankincense, Sandalwood, Benzoin, Ginger.

Immune Stimulants: These oils help to build up immunity and to speed recovery. Good oils in this category include Tea Tree, Geranium, Lavender, Rosemary, Frankincense, and Clove.

Chapter 5:
Diluting the Oils

How to Safely Dilute the Oils and What to Dilute Them In

The one constant is that essential oils should never be applied neat to the skin, with the exception of Lavender and Tea Tree oils. Because essential oil are so concentrated, applying them neat to the skin could result in a negative reaction and damage to your skin.

Fortunately, because the oils are so concentrated, you really do not need much to get the full benefit of the healing effects.

If you are going to be using the essential oils in beauty treatments or in healing remedies, you also need to know how to mix them with the right bases to get the best possible results.

Whilst you can mix essential oils into just about any oily base, there is definitely something to be said for choosing a base that is, in itself, a healing treatment. In this chapter I will speak about blending oils into an aqueous cream base and blending them into a number of different curative oils.

If you do not like the feel of oil on your skin, use a cream base - you can boost its curative properties by blending in some special oils at a 10% concentration - this gives you the benefit of the oils whilst still leaving you with a creamy, lighter texture.

Aqueous Base

An aqueous cream is very simply a cream that has fewer ingredients - it is very moisturizing and is usually not colored or scented. These creams are ideal for people who battle with allergies and sensitive skin.

The bland base cream is ideal to add essential oils to so get yourself a fair amount of it, especially if you are going to start making your own body lotions.

Take some time and source an organic cream - it really is worth paying a bit extra here as the organic-based creams are a lot richer and more nourishing and tend to hold up better than the standard ones.

If you are serious about anti-aging or skin treatments, take the time to get an organic supplier. We have one that is about a half an hours drive away so I buy a liter or two at a time. Our supplier is great - you can take in your old containers for a refill if you like.

Whilst an organic aqueous cream is likely to cost a bit more, it can still prove more cost effective than buying a range of different treatment oils that may go off later. The one my supplier makes is a combination of Sweet Almond oil and Grape Seed oil.

If you really cannot find a supplier, or are keen on DIY creams, you can look up making your own base on the Internet. It is quite a tricky process though and I have found that it is much simpler to buy it ready made. Still, if that is something that interests you, check around online - there are plenty of recipes available.

Whilst I prefer an organic base, I will use an everyday cream at a push. If expense is a problem for you, save the organic cream to use on your face and use the normal stuff on your body. It is not as nourishing but does still provide some moisture and the essential oils added do boost its effectiveness.

I prefer to use a cream base for making day treatments. For night treatments, I stick to cream in spring and summer and an oil base in fall and winter.

Get yourself a few glass jars that have lids that screw on tightly. A shorter jar with a wider mouth is a far better idea in this case - this allows you to scoop out the cream more easily.

It is also a good idea to buy some labels at the same time. I usually look for circular labels that I can put on the bottom of the bottle or the lid of the bottle so that they are less likely to be damaged by oil spilling. Alternatively, cover the labels with clear film and stick it down well. If they do get cream spilled on them, they will turn clear and you will not be able to read the writing on them.

Write your label out as you are making your blend so that you don't forget the ingredients - list the date, the oils used and what the blend is meant to treat. Do take this extra step or you risk ending up with a cupboard full of half-used bottles that you have forgotten the ingredients to.

Also, if a blend works well, you want to be able to duplicate it easily in future.

When it comes to the right dilution of essential oils to cream, it is actually pretty easy to work out - you will use no more than 6 drops of essential oils for each 10ml of cream and this dosage is only to be resorted to in severe cases.

You should only use half this maximum dose when creating a cream for your face as the skin on the face is a lot more delicate.

To be on the safe side, always start at a lower dosage of oils and always do a patch test first before applying them all over. If the oils do not irritate the skin, you may increase the concentration as long as it never exceeds 6 drops for every 10ml of cream.

If there is a reaction and you have used a blend of oils, you may need to test each oil individually to see which one is causing the adverse reaction.

When making your cream, it is important to stir the cream very well so that the oils are completely incorporated. I use a clean paddle stick to do this but a wooden skewer works just as well. If you are using your kitchen utensils, stick to stainless steel ones only - silicone and plastic will absorb the odors of the oils and become unsuitable for use in food preparation.

I normally only make up enough to last a couple of weeks or so, so I don't usually worry about adding preservatives. To prevent bacterial growth in the cream, make sure that the jars are sterilized before use and always clean your hands thoroughly before applying the cream. If this is something that is of concern to you, you can add a capsule of Vitamin E oil for every 250ml of cream used. Vitamin E oil is a natural preservative.

Using a fixative oil like Sandalwood or Cedar Wood is also a good way to preserve the blend naturally.

That said, in twenty or so years I have relied on Sandalwood as a fixative and never really bothered with the Vitamin E. The only time I had a problem with a cream going off was when I added fresh plant matter to the cream - and it was only one out of three batches that went off in that case.

Carrier Oils

In aromatherapy practice, it is more common to blend the oils into a carrier oil. This makes for a more deeply moisturizing treatment overall. If you do not like using oil on your skin, stick to the aqueous cream. It is a commonly held belief that using oil on your skin will cause it to become blocked and spotty but, if you use the right oil, this is a false belief. Grape Seed oil, for example, is a lighter and more toning oil that can help to balance excess sebum in the skin.

The general rule when it comes to choosing a carrier base for use on your skin is that the drier the skin is, the more nourishing the oil that is needed. Sweet Almond oil is a more nourishing oil and can be used on all skin types.

Boost the treatment value of your oil by adding in special treatment oils at a concentration of about 10%. You will often find that the richer oils like Avocado oil have a texture that is unpleasant to use neat on your skin.

If you need a quick massage base oil to use, you can turn to your kitchen cupboards. Sunflower oil does not have a pleasant texture but it is absorbed okay and is quite handy if you need to give someone a quick shoulder rub.

I used to have a very fine rash of bumps on my upper arms - the skin there was very dry and so I blended Olive oil with Neroli oil, Sandalwood oil and Geranium oil. I massaged in morning and evening and the bumps went away. A good quality olive oil is deeply moisturizing and also has anti-bacterial and anti-fungal properties.

I would advise against using either of these oils on the face as they are not refined enough - even when applied to the body there is usually some excess that needs to be wiped away. Here are some of the oils that you may consider instead:

Sweet Almond Oil or Apricot Kernel Oil

These are both from the same family and tend to have similar properties. Both oil are rich in nutrients and suitable for use on all skin types. They are one of the richer oils and so suit those with dry or irritated skin well. They are very soothing to use and will not irritate sensitive skin. If you need to treat eczema, these are the ideal base oils. Use with care or avoid altogether if you have an allergy to nuts.

Sweet Almond oil contains Vitamins A, B1, B2 and B6. The oil does have a small amount of Vitamin E in it and it is a very stable oil to use. This oil lasts well and does not go rancid very quickly. You are typically looking at a shelf-life of around about a year to two years.

Avocado Oil

You may have a choice between refined and unrefined Avocado oil as it is sold both ways. Stick to the refined varieties. Even these are very rich and feel quite heavy. It is said that Avocado oil mimics the skin's own oils almost exactly. Because of the density of the oil, it is better to use it in lower concentrations. If you have severely dry or damaged skin, mix equal quantities of Avocado oil and another oil. For normal day to day use, a 10% - 20% concentration of the oil is more than enough.

Because it has a similar structure to the skin's own, it is fairly easily absorbed. It makes a wonderful anti-aging treatment and is great for healing burned skin and scar tissue.

It contains Vitamins A, B1, B2 and D as well as Lecithin. It does not, unfortunately, keep very well so you should only buy smaller bottles. You are looking at a shelf life of around 6 months to a year in absolutely ideal conditions.

Calendula Oil

Calendula oil is a nourishing oil and promotes skin regeneration. It will help acne heal and prevent further scarring. You can add it into your cream to help heal burns and stretch marks. For a real boost, also add in Hypericum oil.

This oil is good to use on the face and will help to reduce the appearance of thread veins. It can also help to heal varicose veins. It makes a wonderful addition to a cream to moisturize and heal dry, irritated skin that is prone to rashes.

If you suffer with dry eczema, a 10% concentration of Calendula oil applied twice daily will work wonders.

Mix 3-6 drops of Chamomile oil and apply to your cheek over the site of a tooth extraction for pain relief.

This oil contains Vitamins A, B, D and E and is not likely to go rancid too quickly. You are looking at an average shelf life of between 1 and 2 years.

Coconut Oil

Coconut oil became the darling of the health industry a few years ago but it has long been used in beauty treatments to moisturize hair and skin. The oil is solid at room temperature and so makes an excellent base for lip balms and body butters. If you want a more liquid texture, you will need to heat the oil and add equal quantities of another carrier oil.

Coconut oil is absorbed well by the skin and makes it silky smooth and soft. It is a rich oil that can be used on any different skin type. That said, it is known to cause skin rashes so it should be used more sparingly. It is better to get the cold-pressed oil as there is less chance of solvent residue in it.

The oil contains Trimyristin, Caproic Acids and Glycerides and is a very stable oil, even at higher temperatures. You are looking at a shelf-life of 1 - 2 years.

Evening Primrose Oil

This is an oil that contains a high proportion of healing fatty acids and is suitable for use on all skin types. It is especially useful to those with skin that is on the dry and irritated side and it makes a good anti-aging treatment as well. It is often used in blends to treat psoriasis and eczema and is an excellent oil to use to help heal wounds. It can help reduce scarring.

Only Borage oil has a higher concentration of gamma linoleic acid. It also contains oleic acid and linoleic acid in significant quantities as well. This oil lasts well - you have a shelf-life of around 1 - 2 years.

Grape Seed Oil

Sweet Almond oil and Grape Seed oil are the top two choices for aromatherapists because they are very stable oils, have a long shelf life and are well-absorbed by the body.

Grape Seed oil can be used by people with any skin type but benefits those with skins that are oilier and those that have larger pores. The oil is a little lighter than Sweet Almond oil and more astringent.

If you are using Grape Seed oil, make sure that it is the refined variety - the unrefined variety is less expensive but is not recommended for therapeutic use at all.

Grape Seed oil contains Vitamin E and Linoleic acid and lasts very well. It has a shelf-life of around 1 - 2 years.

Hazelnut Oil

This oil is an astringent oil and is suitable for use on oily or combination skin. It is a little too harsh for dry, sensitive skin. It is great for treating acne though. Check whether you are getting pure Hazelnut oil - it is one of the more expensive oils and is often diluted with other oils.

It contains Oleic acid and Linoleic acid and lasts relatively well. It has a shelf-life or around 1 - 1 ½ years.

Jojoba Oil/ Wax

Jojoba is a very popular component of many commercial skin preparations. It is extremely nourishing but does not clog up the pores of the skin. It can help acne to heal and reduce the inflammation present. It reduces scarring.

What is not as well known is that Jojoba is useful in helping reduce inflammation associated with rheumatism and arthritis.

It is more of a wax than an oil as it remains solid at room temperature. If you need a more viscous oil, mix it with equal quantities of a different carrier oil.

It has a large proportion of Vitamin E making it less prone to oxidation. It will last well and you may add it into a blend to help extend the shelf-life of the blend as a whole. It has a shelf-life of around 2 years.

Macadamia Nut

Macadamia Nut oil is one of the best oils for anti-aging. It is suitable for use on any skin type but is particularly helpful to dry, mature skin. Apply daily before going out to boost your skin's natural protection against the sun. It helps restore normal sebum production and is very similar in makeup to the skin's own sebum.

It contains oleic acid and palmitoleic acid. It does not oxidize easily and can be used to extend the shelf-life of any blend. It has a shelf-life or around 2 years.

Wheatgerm Oil

This is a really great oil for anti-aging as it has a high anti-oxidant content. It is best to use it in smaller concentrations - no more than 5% - 10% at a time. The texture and the scent of the oil at higher concentrations can be off-putting.

It is very nourishing for dry and mature skin and helps damaged skin to regenerate. It can assist in clearing up allergic skin reactions.

What is not as well known is that it is also great for loosening up stiff and sore muscles.

If applying to the face, use it no more than twice a week as it can stimulate hair production.

It has high levels of Vitamin E, phytosterols, Vitamin A, Vitamin B Complex and lecithin. It lasts very well due to its high anti-oxidant content and can help to extend the shelf-life of other blends. It has a shelf-life of around 2 years.

Special Treatment Oils

The following oils can be added in need when the skin is in need of a little bit of extra care and a boost. With these oils it is generally better to keep to about 10% concentration and to blend with either Sweet Almond oil or Grape Seed oil.

Borage Oil

Borage oil is highly nourishing and can help to soothe irritated skin. It can be added in very low concentrations to a treat eczema and psoriasis. Use the oil at a maximum concentration of 10%.

Carrot Oil

Can sooth and calm irritated skin.

Castor Oil

Whilst this is quite commonly found in cosmetics, I find that it has a rather unpleasant texture and is quite sticky. That said, if you have an abscess or sore, it can help to fight off infection and help the wound to heal. Apply neat to the area that requires treatment. If you would like to try it in a blend for moisturizing, add no more than 5% concentration. Frankly though, there are much better oils for moisturizing.

Cocoa Butter

This is a nice moisturizing oil but I usually add it in more for the aroma than anything else. If you are on a tight budget, this is not an essential treatment oil.

Lime Blossom Oil

This is a great oil to have on hand. It can help to reduce the appearance of wrinkles, is soothing and relaxing if you have trouble sleeping and can help to relieve pain and swelling if you are arthritic.

Linseed Oil

This has a high proportion of fatty acids and is a great healer and soother. Use in lower concentrations - no more than 10%.

Meadowsweet Oil

If you battle with arthritic or rheumatic pain, this is a good oil to get. Massage in twice daily to help reduce swelling and provide pain relief.

Palm Kernel Oil

This is similar to coconut oil in terms of properties and less likely to cause skin reactions. The actual color of the oil can be a little off-putting and I would advise using a lower concentration of between 5% and 10%.

Peanut Oil

Peanut oil has strong anti-inflammatory properties and can help reduce arthritic pain.

Rosehip Oil

This is one of the best anti-aging treatments and can be used neat on the skin. It has high levels of Vitamin C in it and helps the skin to regenerate. Apply after cleansing the skin and allow to soak in for a few minutes before wiping off residue.

St John's Wort/Hypericum

If you have burnt skin, this is a good oil to have on hand. Mix one part Hypericum oil and one part Calendula oil, add in a drop or two of Geranium oil and a drop of Lavender oil and a drop of Palmarosa oil and the skin will heal much faster.

Chapter 6:
Mommy and Me Time

Essential Oils for Expectant Mothers and Young Children

You can use some essential oils when you are pregnant but you do need to be very careful which oils you choose. An oil such as Rosemary oil, for example, can stimulate the uterus and cause an abortion of the fetus.

If you are trying to fall pregnant or are in your first trimester, I would advise using only the very gentlest of oils - Lavender and Chamomile, unless under the recommendation of a licensed aromatherapist.

Check out any oils that you may like to use and if you do not feel comfortable that it may be safe, leave it out completely.

NEVER Use These Oils if You Are Pregnant

These are dangerous for the baby as they may cause uterine contractions. If you are trying to have a child, think there is a possibility that you are pregnant or have been diagnosed as pregnant don't even think about using these oils:

Basil oil, Clove oil, Cinnamon oil, Myrrh oil, Rosemary oil, Sage oil, Thyme oil. These oils can cause a miscarriage.

In Your Final Trimester

You may add these oils in low concentrations in your final trimester:

Fennel oil, Rose oil, Peppermint oil, Cedar Wood oil.

Again, if you are unsure, just rather leave the oil out altogether.

Stop Stretch Marks from Developing

Carrier Oils:

15ml of Borage oil

15ml of Rose-Hip oil

60ml of Jojoba oil

Essential Oils:

4 Drops Neroli oil

4 Drops Frankincense oil

2 Drops Lavender oil

Mix everything together - any of the essential oils can be exchanged for the others though this blend is particularly effective at reducing the formation and appearance of stretch marks. If you cannot find the Borage oil, substitute with either Rose-Hip or Jojoba oils.

Once you have passed the first trimester, you can also add in 2 drops of Geranium oil to boost this blend even more.

This is also a mix that can help lift your spirits and help you to relax.

Massage gently into the tummy and breast area at least twice a day.

A Less Sweet Blend

Carrier Oils:

15ml of Borage oil

15ml of Rose-Hip oil

60ml of Jojoba oil

Essential Oils:

4 Drops Vetiver oil

4 Drops Sandalwood oil

2 Drops Lavender oil

Also use twice a day. This blend is also great for helping you to relax and will help soothed frayed nerves and sore muscles.

Reducing Anxiety and Depression during Pregnancy

Pregnancy is supposed to be the happiest time of your life but the truth is that it doesn't always feel that way. With hormones in the body raging, your mood can swing from angel to Queen of Evil in a matter of minutes. I once worked with a woman who really battled with pregnancy - she apologized ahead of time because pregnancy turned her into a real witch. Whilst this is an extreme example, having a blend of oils on hand can help to boost mood and help you to feel a little better.

Worries about the change in your body size and shape can be allayed a little by massaging soothing oils into the skin so that at least you need not worry as much about getting stretch marks.

Get your partner in on the action and have them run you a nice warm bath. Add in 2 drops of Neroli oil, 2 Drops of Lavender oil and 2 Drops of Sandalwood oil and feel the anxiety and aches soak away.

Alternatively, blend the same oils into 100ml of Sweet Almond oil and let your partner give you a nice, relaxing shoulder rub.

Vetiver oil is another deeply relaxing essential oil and can re-balance the emotions and stave off stress. Vetiver smells rich and earthy and can be used on its own or in a blend to great success.

Reducing Pregnancy Aches and Pains

As baby grows, he becomes heavier and heavier and your own body starts to ache more and more. Since the Ibuprofen is off the menu, you might want to try some essential oils to help you feel better.

The good news is that Chamomile essential oil is the most effective of all the oils when it comes to pain relief and reducing inflammation and it is gentle enough to be used throughout your pregnancy without fear of complications. Blending it with Lavender oil makes it a highly effective pain killer, a good treatment for skin and a soothing blend for the nerves that will help you sleep better at night.

Sweet Chamomile Blend

Carrier Oils:

20ml Sweet Almond oil

Essential Oils:

3 drops Lavender oil

3 Drops Chamomile oil

Rub into you back or whatever part of your body is aching at least once or twice a day. I often find it useful to follow up the application of the oil with a warm shower. Give the oil about 10 minutes to be absorbed and then have a warm shower. The heat from the shower will help any leftovers sink in and will also help to enhance the relaxing effects of the treatment.

Oil to Help Muscle Aches after the First Trimester

Carrier Oils:

20ml Sweet Almond oil

Essential Oils:

3 drops Vetiver oil

3 Drops Geranium oil

3 Drops Sandalwood oil

Rub into the area at least once or twice a day.

Cold Compress for Relief from Heat and Headaches

If are your biggest in the heat of summer there is good news and bad news - the good news is that you won't be getting up in the freezing cold for nightly feeds. The bad news is that so close to the end of your pregnancy, the hot weather can really make you uncomfortable.

Cool compresses form a double function - they help to physically cool you down and act as a delivery system for the essential oils that you want to use.

You'll need a wash cloth and a bowl of cool water. You add the essential oils to the water and less the wash cloth soak in it. The wash cloth is then wrung out and placed on the back of the neck or on your forehead to help you cool down.

What I sometimes do is to use two wash cloths, soaking the second one while the first is in use. Swap the clothes out when the first has warmed up.

Add the following oils:

2 Drops of Lavender oil

2 Drops of Chamomile oil

1 Drop of Sandalwood oil

1 Drop of Neroli (Optional)

Enjoy Your Pregnancy

If you find that you are prone to blue moods, grab a bottle of Neroli oil and sprinkle a few drops onto a handkerchief or tissue. Sniff repeatedly through the day - keep on hand so that you can get to it easily. My mother told me about this one and she used to stick the tissue in the sleeve of her jersey to keep it easily accessible.

A drop or two of Sandalwood oil will help to reduce feelings of anxiety.

If you are finding that it is tough to cope or feel overwhelmed, also add a drops of Chamomile oil.

If these oils do not appeal to you, Vetiver is a good option from the second trimester onwards - it is relaxing and grounding and not as sweet as the floral oils.

Once you know what oils are safe to use, feel free to experiment a bit. Due to the hormonal changes, a blend that you find wonderful today could leaving you feeling nauseous in a week's time so it is good to have some backups just in case.

Beating Post-Natal Depression

Post-Natal Depression seems so unnatural - how can we be depressed after bringing a new life into the world? It can also make new mothers feel that something is wrong with them. If you consider that a baby means a big life change and that you are sleep deprived as well, it is actually a wonder that more people don't suffer from post-natal depression.

There is nothing wrong with basic post-natal depression, but if you feel as though you are totally overwhelmed or if you feel that you will hurt your child, it is important to get help. The real you would never in a million years do anything to harm your baby but post-natal depression can take on a more sinister side so get help if you need it and don't feel alone - it happens to a lot of new mothers.

2 Drops Neroli oil

2 Drops Lavender oil

2 Drops Ylang Ylang oil

2 Drops Sandalwood oil

Use this in a burner, or add to 20ml of a carrier oil of your choice and massage into skin.

Alternatively, this blend can really help to lift depression:

2 Drops Neroli oil

2 Drops Benzoin oil

2 Drops Cedar Wood oil

Use this in a burner, or add to 20ml of a carrier oil of your choice and massage into skin. Alternatively, add it to you bath water.

Essential Oils and Your Kids

Essential oils can be used for your kids but here you again need to do a little research. Not all oils are suitable to use on kids and you must use the oils that you can use in much lower dilutions than you would on yourself.

It must be remembered that the smaller your child is, the lower the dosage of essential oils must be. Would you, for example, give your baby the same dose of cold medication that you would take? Of course not! The same rule applies to essential oil usage.

Start out by doing a patch test on your skin to make sure that your skin is not irritated by the oil. If your skin tingles, reduce the concentration and repeat until a suitable concentration is reached.

Also do a patch test on your child before dousing them in the oil to make sure that they are not allergic to it at all.

Start with the lowest possible concentration and increase only as necessary. NEVER exceed the maximum doses outlined below unless upon the recommendation of a licensed aromatherapist.

0 - 10 weeks: For the first 10 weeks of his life, baby has enough to contend with and should not be exposed to essential oils. His system at this stage is not strong enough to properly process and excrete the oils and sensitization and toxic buildup could result.

10 weeks - 1 year: No more than 1 drop of essential oil in every 10ml of carrier oil.

1 year - 8 years: No more than 2 drops of essential oil in every 10 ml of carrier oil.

Massage for babies can be a relaxing experience for mother and child. You should not massage baby if they are ill, have just been immunized, have just eaten or are about to eat. Always avoid areas where the skin is broken or where there is new scar tissue.

Always set up in a room that is warm enough for baby and proceed slowly, working your way up from the feet and gently working towards the heart. Use gentle strokes and make sure that baby is enjoying the process. Tug gently to loosen the limbs. Follow off with by wrapping baby in a nice cuddly towel or blanket and have a cuddle. Depending on the oils that you used, this should soon put baby to sleep.

Blend for Skin Conditions in Young Children

1 Drop Chamomile oil

1 Drop Lavender oil

Mix into 20ml of sweet almond oil or a blend of sweet almond and avocado oils (10ml each.) Massage over the whole body, avoiding the genitals. This blend can also help baby sleep.

Blend for Colic in Young Children

1 Drop Mandarin oil or 1 Drop Sweet Orange oil and 1 drop of Lavender oil, mixed into 20ml of a carrier oil of your choice and massaged into the back, chest and abdomen twice a day.

Dealing with Colds and Flu in Young Children

1 Drop Tea Tree oil, 1 Drop Eucalyptus oil and 1 drop of mixed into 30ml of the carrier oil of your choice or placed in a diffuser will help clear up symptoms of colds and flu.

Chapter 7:

Essential Oils for Skin Ailments

Clearing Up Rashes and Other Skin Complaints Naturally

When it comes to the skin, there is a lot that can actually go wrong, allergic reactions can spring up overnight or we can injure ourselves. Even if there is nothing medically wrong, we might end up with skin that is not looking its best. Make-up, pollution and exposure to the elements can also have a negative effect on the skin, especially as we get older.

Fortunately essential oils can help. What follows is a list of conditions that can be treated very effectively using essential oils. For most treatments for the skin, you will apply the oil in either an oil or aqueous base. It is always important, before using a particular oil, that you check that it is suitable for use on your skin. If you have skin that is sensitive, you need to steer clear of any oils that might irritate it.

Remember that the skin on your face is also more delicate than that on the rest of your body. Treat it accordingly. Always do a patch test when using a new oil or blend and always stick to the lowest concentrations of oils that you can find.

In general, the delicate area around the eye needs delicate handling so a lighter cream or oil is called for here.

Anti-Allergy Cream

5 Drops Lavender oil

5 Drops Chamomile oil

100ml Aqueous cream

Mix together all the ingredients well and apply to the affected areas 2 - 3 times a day.

No More Eczema

5 Drops Rose Geranium oil

5 Drops Palmarosa oil

5 Drops Sandalwood oil

5 Drops Lavender oil

200ml Organic aqueous cream

Mix together all the ingredients and apply twice daily to soothe eczema and help to clear it up. The key here is consistency in your treatment.

General Blend for Dry, Flaky Skin

1 Drop Chamomile oil

1 Drop Lavender oil

Mix into 20ml of aqueous cream to which you have added 5ml of Avocado or Helychrisum oil and blend well. Dab on as required.

Heat Rash Blend

2 drops Rose oil

2 drops Chamomile oil

2 drops Lavender oil

50ml Rose Water

Mix all ingredients and shake well. Dab onto rash to relieve itching and discomfort.

Alternatively, mix the same essential oils into plain, cool water and soak a clean wash cloth in the mixture for a few minutes. Wring out the wash cloth and apply as a cool compress to soothe overheated skin.

Psoriasis Cream

5 drops Lavender oil

5 drops Myrrh

5 drops Tea Tree oil

10ml Avocado oil

10ml Borage oil

200ml thick Aqueous cream

Blend together and apply as needed.

Alternatively, you can blend the same essential oils into 200ml Apple Cider Vinegar and dab onto the affected area two to three times a day.

Treating a Boil or Abscess

This is one of the occasions that calls for neat tea tree oil. Apply a drop or two of neat Tea Tree oil to the boil or abscess to promote fast healing and to clear up the infection.

Cold Compresses for Relieving Eczema

A cool compress can be very effective in healing the itch and discomfort associated with eczema. Simply choose your oils and add a drop of each to a bowl of water. Soak a clean wash cloth in the mixture, wring it out and apply as needed. If the child is less than 6 months old, add a drop of Lavender oil and a drop of Chamomile to the water and apply.

If the child is over 6 months oil, add 2 drop of either Lavender or Chamomile and 2 drops of ONE of the following oils:

For weepy eczema: Myrrh or Patchouli

For scaly eczema: Melissa or Rose

For inflamed eczema: Chamomile or Yarrow

For infected eczema: Tea Tree or Lavender.

For Insect Bites, Burns and Stings

It is inevitable that your child will be bitten or stung by some insect or another at some stage or another. In the case of a sting, take a credit card and scrape over the area to remove the stinger (pulling it out will only result in more toxins entering the system). If it is the first time your child has been stung, I advise heading to the emergency room as a precautionary measure, in case they are allergic.

You can treat minor burns at home but for anything more serious, head to the emergency room. For a minor burn, apply a cold compress with 2 drops Lavender oil and 2 drops Chamomile or Geranium oils.

Bites and stings can be itchy and/ or painful and inflamed so, once you have established that your child will not have an allergic reaction, you need to apply oils that have calming properties. Here are some recipes to try:

Compress for Bee Stings/ Itchy Bites

This blend is also extremely useful when it comes to treating sunburn.

5ml Baking Soda

2 drops Lavender oil

2 Drops Chamomile oil

Mix the baking soda in a little water until it forms a paste and then mix that into a bowl of icy water. Add in the oils and then soak a clean wash cloth in the mixture for a couple of minutes. Apply to the area for instant relief.

Soothing Bath for Sunburn

2 drops Lavender oil

2 drops Chamomile oil

100ml milk

50ml Baking Soda

Draw a tepid bath and add the baking soda while the water is being poured to help it to dissolve properly. Mix the oils in the milk and add to the water just before your child gets in. Allow them to soak for at least 15-20 minutes.

Here is some first aid for your skin and examples of oils you could try:

Antiseptics for cuts, insect bites, spots, etc., for example, thyme, sage, eucalyptus, tea tree, clove, lavender and lemon. Lavender and tea tree can be applied neat. The others need to be diluted in a little oil first. Apply at least two to three times a day.

Anti-inflammatory oils for eczema, infected wounds, bumps, bruises, etc., for example, chamomile, lavender and yarrow. Whether you use an oil or a lotion will depend on the condition being treated - for bruises, either is fine; for eczema, it will depend on whether it is weeping or dry - weeping eczema responds better to a light cream, dry will respond better to an oils based treatment. Apply twice a day.

Fungicidal oils for athletes foot, candida, ringworm, etc., for example, lavender, tea tree, myrrh, patchouli and sweet marjoram. Here again, the base that you use is up to you. Lavender and tea tree should be applied neat. Apply the treatment 4-5 times a day and carry on for at least a week after the last lesion has healed to ensure that the fungus has been killed.

Granulation stimulating or cicatrizing (healing) agents for burns, cuts, scars, stretch marks, etc., for example, lavender, chamomile, rose, neroli, frankincense and geranium. When it comes to scars and stretch marks, adding in around about a 5% to 10% concentration of rose hip oil to the final mix can pay great dividends. Oils with a high fatty acid content, like macadamia nut and avocado oil should be part of your blend as well.

Deodorants for excessive perspiration, cleaning wounds, etc., for example, bergamot, lavender, thyme, juniper, cypress, sage, lemongrass. You might be wondering how you use an oil as a deodorant. A great deodorizing treatment is to put a few drops of the oils you choose into a cup of baking soda. Seal the container and mix well. Leave overnight so that the oils can permeate the mix and use the next day, straight after your shower. Reapply as needed.

Insect repellents and parasiticides for lice, fleas, scabies, ticks, mosquitoes, ants, moths, etc., for example, spike lavender, garlic, geranium, citronella, eucalyptus, clove, camphor, cedar wood. When it comes to insects, especially in summer, getting rid of them is hard. I am fairly lucky when it comes to mosquitoes, they don't seem to like the taste of my blood and will rather snack on other people in the room. If you are not so lucky, try burning a citronella candle or diffusing some of the above-mentioned oils. Using in the bath can also be helpful, as can applying them in a cream base to the skin. Just be careful to use a weaker dilution with these oils as some can cause irritation to the skin. Swap out the oils that you use every now and again.

Chapter 8:
Essential Oils for the Muscular System

Clearing Up Muscular Aches and Pains Naturally

The sad fact is that most people deal with pain or illness in some form or another just about every day of their lives. In some cases, the pain is so severe that medication is abused and a tolerance develops leaving fewer and fewer opportunities to find relief.

Fortunately, essential oils can provide significant pain relief. For chronic conditions such as rheumatism, essential oils such as Sweet Marjoram, Melissa, Black Pepper, Eucalyptus, etc. can provide lasting relief.

The idea is to use the treatment as soon as the twinges start. If you want to, you may use the treatments as a prophylactic measure, but should always switch the oils completely after three weeks and use a different set completely for the next three weeks. This prevents your body from building up a tolerance to the oils.

If you have chronic pain, such as that caused by Fibromyalgia, or something similar, take the time to massage your whole limbs and your neck and shoulders every day. Use firm strokes working your way from the extremities and in towards your heart. Climb into a hot shower afterwards to further relieve pain. At least once a week, in place of the shower, climb into a hot bath. If you do not have elevated blood pressure or epilepsy and you are not pregnant, you can add 1 - 2 cups of Epsom Salts to the mix to further ease pain and to help speed toxins out of your system.

Super Pain Reliever

2 Drops Melissa oil

2 Drops Sweet Marjoram oil

2 Drops Chamomile oil

10ml Carrier oil of your choice

10ml Jojoba oil

Blend all ingredients together and massage into affected areas twice daily or as needed.

You can also cut out the carrier oil and Jojoba oil and use these oils in a hot bath instead. If you are not epileptic and do not have high blood pressure, you can also add 2 cups of Epsom Salts to the bath to help relieve pain.

Pain Relieving Soak

2 Drops Sweet Orange oil

2 Drops Eucalyptus oil

2 Drops Juniper oil

10ml Sweet Almond oil

2 Cups Epsom Salts

½ Cup Baking Soda

Run a bath as hot as you can manage and add in the Epsom Salts and Baking Soda and stir to incorporate. Once your bath is drawn, and just before you get in, mix together the essential oils with the Sweet Almond oil and add to the bath water. Soak for at least 20 minutes.

When you get out of the bath, give yourself a vigorous rub-down with the towel and then wrap up warmly. Sit quietly and relax or climb into bed and sleep. You may feel a little drained after the bath but you will sleep extremely well and will wake up feeling a lot better with fewer aches and pains.

The reason that the treatment makes you feel drained is that it is has a strong detoxifying action.

This treatment is not suitable for pregnant women, people with high blood pressure or epileptics.

A Less Drastic Treatment Option

It is not always convenient to soak in a hot bath, especially if you have high blood pressure or are pregnant. For muscle aches, it is recommended that you apply the oils to the skin, in a suitable base - here diffusion will not help. A few drops in the bath or even just a foot bath might do the trick, but a nice rub with a blend of oils is the best bet for muscular pain.

Personally I find the blend above very soothing - instead of applying it and then bathing, climb into a hot shower or just leave it to soak in.

 Another great muscle relaxant, and one that I really do love, is Vetiver oil and sandalwood oil. This is especially great for when you are feeling completely stressed out and full of nervous tension.

If you have a long day ahead of you and are battling with muscular aches, mix together equal quantities of Eucalyptus oil, Peppermint oil and Sweet Orange oil and massage into affected areas. This treatment is not suitable to use at night time as the Peppermint has a stimulating effect on the mind.

Here are some other oils for you to try out when dealing with muscular pain:

Antispasmodics for menstrual cramp (dysmenorrhea), labor pains, etc., for example, sweet marjoram, chamomile, Clary sage, jasmine, and lavender. Mix in a suitable base and apply directly to the areas concerned. I have not needed to take pain pills for menstrual cramps in the last 20 years thanks to sweet marjoram oil and lavender. I mix a few drops of each into a base oil and apply as soon as the first twinge starts. If you are really in pain, apply the oils and then put a heat pack on as well.

Uterine tonics and regulators for pregnancy, excess menstruation (menorrhagia), PMT, etc., for example, Clary sage, jasmine, rose, myrrh, frankincense, lemon balm. Some of these oils contain estrogenic compounds that are useful for helping to balance hormones. Again, if this is a regular problem, see your gynecologist. If you are pregnant, always make sure that any oils that you use are suitable for use during pregnancy.

Chapter 9:
Essential Oils for the Nervous System

The Guide to a Calmer and More Focused You

Using oils that you love the smell of and that have good associations for you on a day to day basis will help to improve your mood. When testing oils or blends, it is a good idea to analyze how they affect you emotionally as well checking what the benefits to using them are.

Ideally speaking, find a few different oils that make you feel happier and brighter - Bergamot, Neroli, Rose and Jasmine are just some examples of such oils. Now start using them in your day to day life.

This could be as simple as diffusing the oils. If you are in an office environment and this is not allowed, there are a couple of things that you can do - make a basic hand cream using the essential oil blends of choice. (Just be careful not to use photo-toxic oils if you are going out into the sun.)

Alternatively you can carry a handkerchief sprinkled with the oils and inhale them every now and again. The oils won't last all day so you will need to add more oils.

The simplest alternative by far is to get hold of an opaque plastic or glass bottle with a tight-fitting lid. Either place some tissues or some cotton wool into the bottle, sprinkle on two or three drops of essential oil and seal. Every time you open the bottle, you will get that wonderful, uplifting scent coming out at you.

Keep the bottle in your office drawer or, at a push, your car. That way when you are having a really bad day at work there is a remedy close to hand.

The bottle prevents the essential oils from evaporating too quickly and so you only need to top up the oils once every one or two months.

A great alternative is a roller stick. You may have to buy one with oils in already as these are not that easy to get unused if you are only buying one or two bottles. Once the oils have been finished, lever out the ball section of the lid, rinse well and add your own carrier oils and essential oils.

Making yourself happier through essential oils is quite easy - start incorporating the oils that make you feel good into your personal skin care routine, into your final rinse water when doing washing, etc.

Switch out the oils every once in a while so that you do not develop a tolerance for them.

Happy Day Blend

2 Drops Jasmine oil

2 Drops Benzoin oil

2 Drops Neroli oil

Mix oils together and diffuse them in whatever way seems best to you. Allow at least one hour of exposure a day for a week to see really good results.

Frazzled Nerve Blend

2 Drops Frankincense oil

2 Drops Sandalwood oil

2 Drops Neroli oil

Blend all the oils together and diffuse them for at least 1 hour to get ultimate results. This blend is extremely relaxing and so is good to use during the evening. It is also a good blend to use if you want to meditate.

Come On Get Happy Blend

2 Drops Bergamot oil

2 Drops Jasmine oil

2 Drops Neroli oil

2 Drops Sandalwood oil

Mix oils together and diffuse them in whatever way seems best to you. Allow at least one hour of exposure a day for a week to see really good results.

If it more that you are fatigued rather than actually depressed, you can start using essential oils that stimulate the mind and senses to help you make it through each day.

Fresh smelling oils such as Camphor, Rosemary, Basil, Peppermint and Eucalyptus can help you to shake off fatigue and allow you to get through the day at work.

Once you are home, make sure that there is a cut-off point when work stops completely. After this point there is no checking business emails, writing reports, etc.

Start winding down for bed at least an hour before you want to sleep. Switch off the TV, smart phone and computer and choose relaxing oils such as Chamomile, Vetiver, Sandal wood and Melissa. Diffuse a relaxing blend for about an hour before bedtime to help you sleep really, really well. Spend the time doing something relaxing like reading or knitting and put a nice relaxing CD on to play.

Mix feel-good oils into an aqueous base and make a point of rubbing them into your hands, forearms and elbows every evening - your skin will start to look better and you will feel better as well.

Essential oils that are good for dealing with depression and a low mood include Benzoin, Neroli oil, Bergamot oil, Chamomile oil.

Need to put a bit of a spark back in the sex life? The following oils will help with this goal: Black pepper oil, Cardamom oil, Clary Sage oil, Neroli oil, Jasmine oil, Rose oil, Sandalwood oil, Patchouli oil and Ylang Ylang oil.

Oils to help you sleep include: Chamomile oil, Bergamot, Sandalwood oil, Lavender oil, Sweet Marjoram oil, Lemon Balm oil, Hops oil, Valerian oil, Lemon oil.

Oils that can help you recover from periods of stress and nervous fatigue include, Basil oil, Jasmine oil, Peppermint oil, Ylang Ylang oil, Neroli oil, Angelica oil, Rosemary oil.

Oils that support the nervous system include Chamomile oil, Clary Sage oil, Juniper oil, Lavender oil, Sweet Marjoram oil, Rosemary oil.

Adrenal stimulants for anxiety, stress-related conditions, etc., for example, basil, geranium, rosemary, borneol, sage, pine, savory. These can help you overcome the initial stages of burnout and allow you to carry on working. It is advisable though, to also look into ways to actively manage your stress in a healthy manner as essential oils will not always be able to do this for you.

Chapter 10:

Essential Oils for the Genito-Urinary System

For When There Is A Problem Down There

Men and women alike are often embarrassed to deal with issues in the genito-urinary system and generally prefer to try and deal with the problem themselves before consulting a doctor. If the infection is not clearing after a few days, it is important to see your doctor or risk creating more problems.

I do advocate using essential oils but I also urge caution. For women, a disrupted menstrual cycle is a symptom of something else that has gone wrong, it is not natural, so it is important to visit your gynecologist so that they can rule out any serious issues before you start any natural treatment.

For the more minor issues, here are some oils that you can try:

Antispasmodics for menstrual cramp (dysmenorrhea), labor pains, etc., for example, sweet marjoram, chamomile, Clary sage, jasmine, and lavender.

Emmenagogues for scanty periods, lack of periods (amenorrhea), etc., for example, chamomile, fennel, hyssop, juniper, sweet marjoram, peppermint.

Uterine tonics and regulators for pregnancy, excess menstruation (menorrhagia), PMT, etc., for example, Clary sage, jasmine, rose, myrrh, frankincense, lemon balm.

Antiseptic and bactericidal agents for leucorrhoea, vaginal pruritus, thrush, etc., for example, bergamot, chamomile, myrrh, rose, tea tree. These are best treated using a few drops of the oil in a bath of tepid water or, if mixed into a

Galactagogues for increasing milk flow; for example, fennel, jasmine, anise, lemongrass (sage, mint and parsley reduce it).

Aphrodisiacs for impotence and frigidity, etc., for example, black pepper, cardamom, Cary sage, neroli, jasmine, rose, sandalwood, patchouli, ylang ylang.

Anaphrodisiacs for reducing sexual desire; for example, sweet marjoram, camphor.

Bathing and using a douche can help control urinary infections, especially when they are associated with nervous or stress-related symptoms.

Urinary antiseptics for cystitis, urethritis, etc., for example, bergamot, chamomile, tea tree, sandalwood.

Chapter 11:

Essential Oils for the Digestive System

Improving Digestion and Relieving Discomfort

When you have an upset tummy, reaching for antacids is not going to be necessary anymore. Essential oils are great for treating indigestion and stomach aches and pains. In fact, any abdominal cramps, even ones caused by menstruation can be eased by using essential oils.

I find that it is easiest to simply mix the oils up in some base oil and to rub them in. Chamomile oil and Lavender oil in equal quantities in a simple sweet almond oil base is my go to treatment for when I have indigestion or cramping. Simply massage the oils in and apply a heat pad for instant relief.

Peppermint oil and Fennel oil are two other really good treatments when it comes to digestive upsets. If you have had a really rich meal, rub on a blend containing one of these two oils to help soothe digestion and prevent acid reflux.

If you are suffering from nausea, Peppermint oil or Ginger oil are a better bet than Chamomile oil.

Here are some oils that you can try for yourself:

Antispasmodics for spasm, pain, indigestion, etc., for example, chamomile, caraway, fennel, orange, peppermint, lemon balm, aniseed, cinnamon.

Carminatives and stomachics for flatulent dyspepsia, aerophagia, nausea, etc., for example, angelica, basil, fennel, chamomile, peppermint, mandarin.

Cholagogues for increasing the flow of bile and stimulating the gall bladder; for example, caraway, lavender, peppermint and borneol.

Hepatics for liver congestion, jaundice, etc., for example, lemon, lime, rosemary, peppermint.

Aperitifs for loss of appetite, anorexia, etc., for example, aniseed, angelica, orange, ginger, garlic.

Conclusion

Thank you again for downloading this book!

I do hope that this book was a great introduction to the world of aromatherapy for you and that you will be able to use the knowledge learned to help make your life and that of your family's healthy and better.

The next step is to actually get going making your own blends and taking full advantage of Mother Nature's pharmacy.

I'd like to ask for one small favor, if you don't mind - please take the time to share your thoughts and post a review on Amazon. I would really appreciate it!

Thank you and good luck!

Made in the USA
Las Vegas, NV
16 November 2021